MW00873661

Prostate Cancer and Sexuality

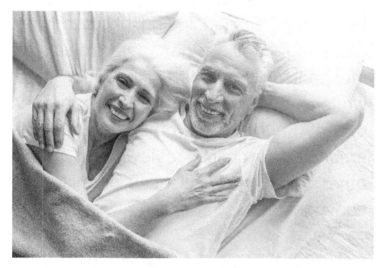

Overcoming Challenges and Enhancing Intimacy

Sawyer Jones

PROSTATE CANCER
AND
SEXUALITY

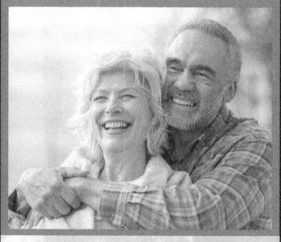

OVERCOMING CHALLENGES
AND ENHANCING INTIMACY

SAWYER JONES

Looking for more information on the diagnosis, treatment, and recovery process for prostate cancer? Check out our companion guide, Prostate Cancer: From Diagnosis to Recovery, which provides in-depth insights and practical advice for men and their loved ones facing prostate cancer. Click here or the cover below to access the book and learn more about navigating the prostate cancer journey."

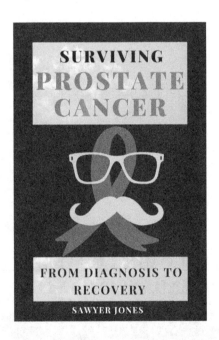

You can also click on the image and you will be directed to the book.

Table of content

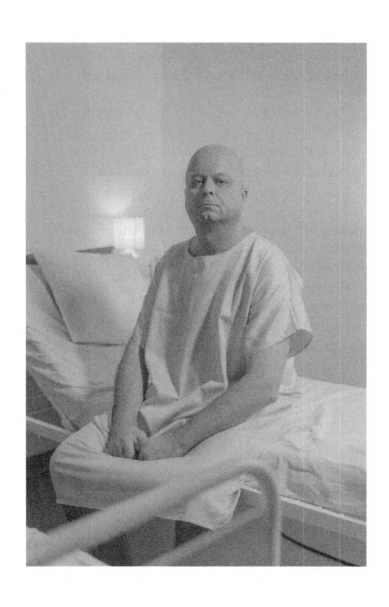

Introduction

As I sat in the urologist's office, waiting for the results of my prostate biopsy, I couldn't help but feel anxious. My mind raced with thoughts of what could be, and I couldn't shake the feeling that something was wrong. When the doctor finally walked in and delivered the news that I had prostate cancer, my world came crashing down.

In the following months, I underwent surgery and radiation treatments to rid my body of cancer. It was a difficult journey, filled with physical and emotional challenges. But with the support of my loved ones and healthcare team, I emerged victorious.

As I entered the recovery phase, I couldn't help but feel grateful for the opportunity to start afresh. However, I soon discovered that the effects of prostate cancer lingered on long after treatment had ended. One of the most significant impacts it had on my life was on my sexual health. I struggled with intimacy and the thought of never experiencing sexual pleasure again.

It was through my own experiences that I realized the need for a book that would help prostate cancer survivors navigate the challenges of sexual health. This led me to write "Prostate Cancer and Sexuality: Overcoming Challenges and Enhancing Intimacy," a guide that provides practical advice and strategies for those struggling with sexual dysfunction after prostate cancer.

In this book, I share my own story and the stories of other prostate cancer survivors who have navigated the challenges of sexual health. I offer tips on how to communicate with healthcare providers, manage sexual dysfunction and incontinence, and enhance intimacy with your partner. I also explore alternative and complementary therapies that may help improve sexual function.

I hope this book will serve as a beacon of hope for all those who have faced the challenges of prostate cancer and sexual dysfunction. Remember, you are not alone, and there is help and support available to you. Let's prioritize our sexual health and embrace a new normal together.

The impact of prostate cancer on sexual health

For many men, prostate cancer brings about significant changes to their sexual health. As a survivor of prostate cancer myself, I can attest to the impact this disease can have on one's intimate relationships. Prior to my diagnosis, I had never considered how my sexual health might be affected by a cancer diagnosis. But after my treatment, I found myself struggling to regain the intimacy and pleasure that I once took for granted.

The reality is that prostate cancer and its treatments can significantly impact sexual health in a number of ways. Whether it's erectile dysfunction, incontinence, or other sexual dysfunctions, these issues can be difficult to talk about and can have a profound impact on one's self-esteem, relationships, and overall quality of life.

That's why I felt it was important to write this book. I want to help other prostate cancer survivors navigate the complex and often challenging landscape of sexual health after cancer. With the right knowledge, tools, and support, it is possible to overcome the challenges and enhance intimacy. I hope this book serves as a resource and guide for all those who are looking to reclaim their sexual health and maintain a fulfilling and satisfying intimate life after prostate cancer.

The need for addressing sexual health after prostate cancer

After a prostate cancer diagnosis and subsequent treatment, many men experience changes in their sexual health. Sexual dysfunction, such as erectile dysfunction and decreased libido, can be common side effects of treatment. Additionally, incontinence can also affect sexual health, making some men hesitant to engage in sexual activity.

Despite these challenges, addressing sexual health after prostate cancer is essential. Sexuality and intimacy are important parts of overall health and well-being, and can play a significant role in mental and emotional health. By addressing sexual health concerns after prostate cancer treatment, men and their partners can maintain physical intimacy and emotional connection, leading to improved quality of life.

Furthermore, many men may feel embarrassed or ashamed to discuss their sexual health concerns with healthcare providers or partners. However, addressing these concerns openly and honestly can lead to better communication, increased support, and improved outcomes. This book aims to provide practical advice and strategies for overcoming the challenges of prostate cancer treatment and enhancing intimacy and sexual function.

The objective of the book

The objective of this book is to provide prostate cancer survivors and their partners with the knowledge and tools necessary to overcome the challenges of sexual dysfunction and enhance their intimacy after prostate cancer treatment. Through a comprehensive guide that covers the physical and psychological impacts of prostate cancer treatment on sexual health, communication with healthcare providers, strategies for improving sexual function and intimacy, and alternative and complementary therapies, this book aims to empower survivors and their partners to take an active role in addressing their sexual health concerns. By highlighting the importance of prioritizing sexual health after prostate cancer, this book seeks to help survivors and their partners move forward with confidence, embracing a new normal and finding new ways to experience pleasure and intimacy.

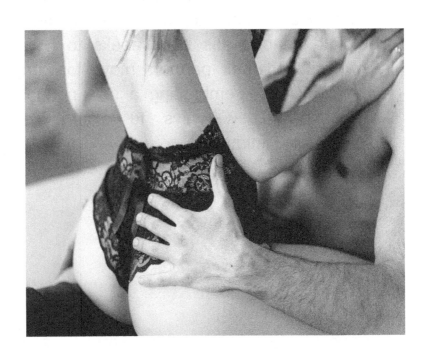

Chapter 1: Understanding Prostate Cancer and Sexual Health

Understanding prostate cancer

Prostate cancer is a common form of cancer that affects the prostate gland in men. The prostate gland is a small walnut-shaped gland located just below the bladder and in front of the rectum. It produces the fluid that carries sperm during ejaculation.

Prostate cancer occurs when cells in the prostate gland grow and multiply uncontrollably, forming a tumor. If the cancer is not treated early, it can spread beyond the prostate gland to other parts of the body, such as the bones and lymph nodes.

There are different types of prostate cancer, including adenocarcinoma (the most common type), sarcoma, small cell carcinoma, and transitional cell carcinoma. The majority of prostate cancers are adenocarcinomas, which start in the cells that produce prostate fluid.

Prostate cancer is the second most common cancer in men worldwide, and the most common cancer in men in the United States. It is estimated that one in eight men will be diagnosed with prostate cancer in their lifetime.

The anatomy of the prostate gland

The prostate gland is a small, walnut-shaped gland located below the bladder and in front of the rectum in men. It surrounds the urethra, which is the tube that carries urine and semen out of the body. The prostate gland is responsible for producing and secreting fluid that nourishes and protects sperm. This fluid is mixed with sperm to form semen, which is ejaculated during sexual activity.

The prostate gland is a small, walnut-shaped gland located below the bladder and in front of the rectum in men. It surrounds the urethra, which is the tube that carries urine from the bladder to the outside of the body. The prostate gland produces and secretes fluid that forms part of the semen, the fluid that carries sperm during ejaculation.

The prostate gland is made up of several types of cells, including glandular cells, which produce the fluid that makes up semen, and stromal cells, which provide structural support to the gland. The gland is also surrounded by a layer of tissue called the capsule, which helps to keep it in place and provides a barrier between the gland and the surrounding tissues.

The prostate gland is an important part of the male reproductive system, but it can also be affected by disease, including prostate cancer. Understanding the anatomy of the prostate gland is important in understanding how prostate cancer can impact sexual health.

The role of the prostate gland in sexual function

The prostate gland plays a crucial role in sexual function, particularly in the production of semen. During sexual arousal, the prostate gland produces a milky fluid that mixes with sperm from the testicles to form semen. This fluid helps to nourish and protect the sperm, as well as provide lubrication during ejaculation.

Additionally, the prostate gland is responsible for regulating the flow of urine through the urethra, which is the tube that carries urine from the bladder to the outside of the body. The prostate surrounds the urethra and produces a fluid that helps to flush out any urine that may be left in the urethra after urination.

Problems with the prostate gland, such as prostate cancer, can significantly impact sexual function and urinary function. Treatment for prostate cancer, such as surgery or radiation therapy, can damage the prostate gland and surrounding tissues, leading to sexual dysfunction and urinary incontinence.

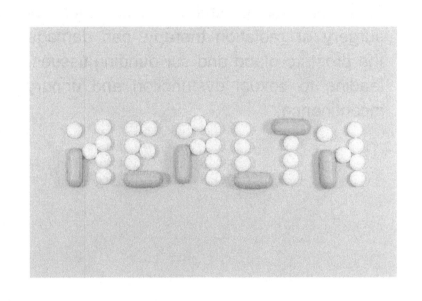

Chapter 2: The Effects of Prostate Cancer Treatment on Sexual Health

Types of prostate cancer treatment

There are several types of treatment options for prostate cancer, including:

Watchful waiting or active surveillance: This approach involves monitoring the cancer for any changes without immediately starting treatment.

Surgery: This involves the removal of the prostate gland and some surrounding tissue.

Radiation therapy: This treatment uses high-energy rays to kill cancer cells.

Hormone therapy: This treatment aims to stop or slow down the growth of cancer cells by blocking the effects of male hormones such as testosterone.

Chemotherapy: This treatment uses drugs to kill cancer cells.

Immunotherapy: This treatment stimulates the body's immune system to fight cancer cells.

Bone-directed therapy: This treatment is used to prevent or treat bone metastasis (when cancer spreads to the bones) and includes medications such as bisphosphonates and denosumab.

The type of treatment recommended by your doctor will depend on several factors, including the stage and grade of your cancer, your overall health and personal preferences. It is important to discuss the potential risks and benefits of each treatment option with your healthcare provider.

The impact of prostate cancer treatment on sexual health

Prostate cancer treatment can have a significant impact on a man's sexual health. The most common treatments for prostate cancer, such as surgery, radiation therapy, and hormone therapy, can cause a range of sexual side effects that can last for months or even years.

One of the most common sexual side effects of prostate cancer treatment is erectile dysfunction (ED), which is the inability to achieve or maintain an erection firm enough for sexual intercourse. Surgery to remove the prostate gland, known as a prostatectomy, can damage the nerves that control erections, leading to ED. Radiation therapy can also damage the blood vessels and nerves that support erections, causing ED. Hormone therapy, which works by reducing the level of testosterone in the body, can also cause ED.

In addition to ED, prostate cancer treatment can also cause other sexual side effects, such as a decrease in libido, or sex drive, and a decrease in the intensity of orgasms. Some men may also experience difficulty ejaculating or experience pain during ejaculation.

The impact of these sexual side effects can be significant, affecting a man's self-esteem, his sense of masculinity, and his relationships with his partner. Many men feel embarrassed or ashamed to talk about their sexual side effects, which can lead to feelings of isolation and depression.

It's important for men to know that they are not alone in experiencing sexual side effects after prostate cancer treatment. Healthcare providers can offer a range of treatments and strategies to manage these side effects, including medications, vacuum erection devices, penile injections, and counseling.

It's also important for men to talk openly with their partner about their sexual concerns and to explore different ways of being intimate, such as cuddling, touching, and other forms of physical affection. By working together and seeking help when needed, men and their partners can find ways to maintain a fulfilling and satisfying sex life after prostate cancer treatment.

The physical effects of prostate cancer treatment on sexual function

Prostate cancer treatment can have significant physical effects on sexual function. Surgery and radiation therapy are the most common treatments for prostate cancer, and both can cause damage to the nerves and blood vessels that are necessary for erections. The nerves that control erections run along the sides of the prostate gland, and both surgical and radiation treatments can damage these nerves.

Surgery for prostate cancer, known as a prostatectomy, involves the removal of the entire prostate gland, including the seminal vesicles and some of the surrounding tissue. This can cause damage to the nerves and blood vessels responsible for erections, leading to difficulty achieving or maintaining an erection. This is known as erectile dysfunction.

Radiation therapy for prostate cancer also has the potential to damage the nerves and blood vessels involved in erections. Radiation can cause inflammation and scarring of the tissue around the prostate gland, which can lead to erectile dysfunction.

In addition to erectile dysfunction, prostate cancer treatment can also cause other physical effects on sexual function, such as reduced semen volume and changes in orgasm intensity. Radiation therapy can cause irritation of the bladder and urethra, leading to painful urination and difficulty achieving orgasm.

It's important to note that not all men experience the same physical effects of prostate cancer treatment on sexual function. Some men may experience only mild or temporary changes, while others may experience more severe or permanent changes. It's also possible for sexual function to improve over time, especially with the help of treatment and lifestyle changes.

If you're experiencing physical effects of prostate cancer treatment on your sexual function, it's important to talk to your healthcare provider. There are treatments and therapies available that can help manage these effects and improve sexual function.

The psychological effects of prostate cancer treatment on sexual function

Prostate cancer treatment can have a significant impact on a man's mental health and emotional wellbeing, including his sexual function. Men may experience a range of psychological effects as a result of their treatment, such as:

Anxiety: Men may feel anxious about the impact of their treatment on their sexual function and may worry about whether they will be able to perform sexually after treatment.

Depression: Prostate cancer treatment can cause changes in hormone levels, which can contribute to depression. Men may also feel depressed due to the physical side effects of treatment and the impact on their sexual function.

Loss of confidence: Changes in sexual function can lead to a loss of confidence and self-esteem, which can affect a man's overall quality of life.

Relationship issues: Prostate cancer treatment can also affect a man's intimate relationships, leading to feelings of guilt, shame, and isolation. Partners may also struggle to understand and cope with the changes in sexual function.

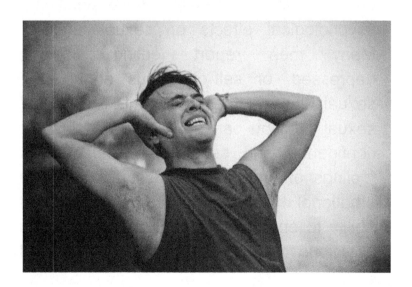

It is important for men to be aware of these potential psychological effects and to seek support from their healthcare providers, loved ones, and mental health professionals if needed. Counseling, support groups, and other resources are available to help men cope with the emotional and psychological impact of prostate cancer treatment on their sexual function and overall wellbeing.

In addition to the physical effects, prostate cancer treatment can also have significant psychological effects on sexual function. Many men report feeling anxious, depressed, or self-conscious about their sexual function after treatment. The loss of sexual function can also lead to a loss of confidence and self-esteem, as well as feelings of shame or emasculation. These emotional effects can further impact a man's ability to engage in sexual activity, creating a vicious cycle of physical and emotional distress.

It's important to note that the psychological effects of prostate cancer treatment on sexual function are not limited to the patient alone. Partners may also experience emotional distress and feelings of loss, as they navigate changes to their sexual relationship. Communication and support are key to managing the psychological impact of prostate cancer treatment on sexual health, for both the patient and their partner.

Fortunately, there are strategies and resources available to help men and their partners cope with the psychological effects of prostate cancer treatment on sexual function. Seeking support from a mental health professional, joining a support group, and having open and honest communication with one's healthcare provider and partner are all important steps in managing the emotional impact of prostate cancer treatment on sexual health.

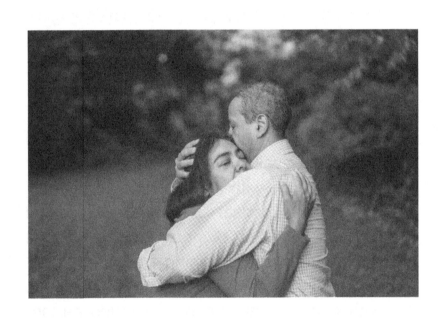

Chapter 3: Communicating with Your Healthcare Provider

Effective communication with your healthcare provider is essential when it comes to addressing sexual health concerns after prostate cancer treatment. It is normal to feel nervous or embarrassed about discussing sexual issues with your doctor, but keep in mind that they are medical professionals who are there to help you. Being open and honest with them about your concerns can help them provide you with the best possible care.

Here are some tips for communicating with your healthcare provider about sexual health concerns:

Be open and honest: It is important to be truthful about any sexual problems you may be experiencing, even if it may be uncomfortable to discuss. Remember that your healthcare provider has heard it all before, and they are there to help you.

Be specific: When discussing sexual issues, be specific about the symptoms you are experiencing, when they started, and how they are affecting your life. This can help your doctor make an accurate diagnosis and recommend appropriate treatment options.

Ask questions: Don't be afraid to ask your healthcare provider questions about your sexual health. Ask about any side effects of treatment, potential treatment options, and any concerns you may have.

Bring a partner: If you have a partner, consider bringing them to the appointment. They can provide valuable input and support during the discussion.

Consider seeking help from a specialist: If you feel uncomfortable discussing sexual health concerns with your primary care doctor, consider seeking help from a specialist. A urologist, for example, is a doctor who specializes in treating conditions of the urinary tract and male reproductive system, and can provide specific expertise in managing sexual health concerns.

Remember, effective communication with your healthcare provider is key in addressing sexual health concerns after prostate cancer treatment. Don't hesitate to speak up and seek the help you need.

Why communication is important

Communication is essential in all aspects of life, and this holds true when it comes to discussing sexual health concerns with your healthcare provider. For men who have undergone treatment for prostate cancer, sexual dysfunction can be a significant issue. It is essential to communicate any problems with sexual health to your healthcare provider to ensure the best possible care and management of the issue.

Effective communication with your healthcare provider can help you to better understand the impact of prostate cancer treatment on your sexual health. It can also help you to identify any potential treatments or therapies that may help to manage any sexual dysfunction or incontinence that may occur. Additionally, communication can help to reduce any feelings of isolation or shame that you may be experiencing, allowing you to address these issues head-on with the help of a medical professional.

Communication can also help to facilitate better care from your healthcare provider. By being open and honest about any sexual health concerns you may have, your healthcare provider can develop a more comprehensive care plan that addresses your unique needs and concerns. This can lead to better outcomes and a higher quality of life for prostate cancer survivors.

Overall, communication is crucial when it comes to addressing sexual health concerns after prostate cancer treatment. It can help to reduce stigma, increase understanding, and lead to better care and management of any sexual dysfunction or incontinence.

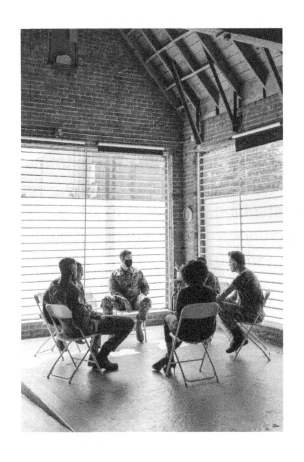

Tips for communicating with your healthcare provider about sexual health concerns

Communicating with your healthcare provider about sexual health concerns can be uncomfortable and difficult. However, it is important to have open and honest conversations with your provider in order to receive the best care possible. Here are some tips for effectively communicating with your healthcare provider about sexual health concerns:

Prepare ahead of time: Before your appointment, make a list of any questions or concerns you have about your sexual health. This will help you stay organized and ensure that you don't forget anything important.

Use clear language: Be specific and clear about your symptoms or concerns. Use language that your healthcare provider will understand, but don't be afraid to use medical terms if you know them.

Be honest: It can be difficult to talk about sexual issues, but it's important to be honest with your healthcare provider. They are there to help you, and they won't judge you or think less of you because of your concerns.

Don't be afraid to ask questions: If you don't understand something your healthcare provider says, ask them to explain it in simpler terms. It's important that you fully understand your condition and your treatment options.

Bring a support person: If you feel uncomfortable discussing your sexual health concerns alone, consider bringing a trusted friend or family member with you to your appointment.

Remember, your healthcare provider is there to help you. By communicating openly and honestly with them about your sexual health concerns, you can receive the care and support you need.

Questions to ask your healthcare provider about sexual health

Here are some questions that you may want to ask your healthcare provider about sexual health after prostate cancer treatment:

- **What types of sexual problems should I expect after my treatment?**
- **How long should I expect these problems to last?**
- **Are there any medications or treatments that can help with my sexual function?**
- **Can I continue to have sexual activity during treatment or recovery?**
- **Are there any risks to having sexual activity after treatment?**
- **Are there any exercises or physical therapy that can help with sexual function?**
- **Are there any lifestyle changes that can help with sexual function?**

- Are there any support groups or resources for sexual health after prostate cancer treatment?
- How often should I follow up with my healthcare provider about my sexual health?
- Are there any additional tests or evaluations that I should undergo to monitor my sexual health?

Feel free to add more…….

Remember that open communication with your healthcare provider is essential for addressing sexual health concerns after prostate cancer treatment. Don't be afraid to ask questions or express your concerns, as your provider is there to help you navigate this important aspect of your recovery.

Chapter 4: Dealing with Sexual Dysfunction and Incontinence

Dealing with sexual dysfunction and incontinence is one of the most challenging aspects of recovering from prostate cancer treatment. While many men can experience a return to normal sexual function after treatment, others may experience long-term sexual dysfunction or incontinence.

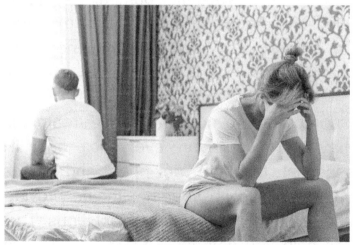

Sexual dysfunction can manifest in various ways, including erectile dysfunction, decreased libido, and difficulty achieving orgasm. Incontinence, on the other hand, refers to the loss of bladder control and can result in urinary leakage or the need to use incontinence pads.

Fortunately, there are strategies for managing and treating sexual dysfunction and incontinence. Your healthcare provider may recommend medications or devices to assist with erectile dysfunction, such as oral medications, vacuum pumps, or penile injections. Additionally, pelvic floor exercises or surgery may be recommended for incontinence.

It's important to note that these treatments may not work for everyone, and it's essential to have an open and honest conversation with your healthcare provider about your concerns and expectations. They can help you determine the best course of action for your individual situation.

In addition to medical treatments, there are also practical strategies for addressing sexual dysfunction and incontinence. For example, using incontinence pads or practicing timed voiding can help manage urinary leakage. And when it comes to sexual function, it's important to explore new ways of intimacy and pleasure that may not involve traditional sexual intercourse.

It's important to remember that sexual dysfunction and incontinence are common side effects of prostate cancer treatment, and there is no shame in seeking help or support. Many men find that support groups or counseling can be helpful in coping with the physical and emotional effects of these conditions.

Understanding sexual dysfunction and incontinence

Sexual dysfunction and incontinence are common issues that affect men after prostate cancer treatment. These conditions can have a significant impact on a man's quality of life and intimate relationships.

Sexual dysfunction can refer to a variety of problems that affect a man's ability to achieve or maintain an erection or ejaculate. This can include erectile dysfunction, decreased libido, and problems with orgasm. These issues can be caused by damage to the nerves and blood vessels that control sexual function during prostate cancer treatment.

Incontinence, on the other hand, refers to the loss of bladder control. This can manifest as leakage of urine or the complete inability to control urination. Incontinence can be caused by damage to the muscles and nerves that control the bladder during prostate cancer treatment.

Both sexual dysfunction and incontinence can be distressing and challenging to manage, but there are strategies and treatments that can help men cope with these issues and improve their quality of life.

Managing sexual dysfunction and incontinence

Managing sexual dysfunction and incontinence after prostate cancer treatment requires a combination of medical intervention, lifestyle changes, and emotional support. Here are some strategies that may help:

Medical interventions: Depending on the severity of the sexual dysfunction or incontinence, your healthcare provider may recommend medication or surgery to manage the symptoms. There are also devices such as penile implants, vacuum pumps, and urethral inserts that can help with erectile dysfunction or incontinence.

Pelvic floor exercises: Pelvic floor muscles play an important role in sexual function and urinary control. Pelvic floor exercises, such as Kegels, can help strengthen these muscles and improve sexual function and incontinence. Your healthcare provider or a physical therapist can guide you on how to perform these exercises correctly.

Lifestyle changes: Lifestyle changes such as quitting smoking, reducing alcohol consumption, and maintaining a healthy weight can help improve sexual function and incontinence. Regular exercise can also improve blood flow to the pelvic area, which can benefit sexual function.

Emotional support: Coping with sexual dysfunction and incontinence can be challenging, and it's important to seek emotional support from loved ones, support groups, or a mental health professional. It's important to communicate openly with your partner about your sexual health concerns and work together to find ways to maintain intimacy.

It's essential to consult with your healthcare provider to determine the best approach for managing sexual dysfunction and incontinence after prostate cancer treatment. They can help identify the underlying cause of the symptoms and recommend appropriate treatment options.

Tips for addressing sexual dysfunction and incontinence with your partner

Sexual dysfunction and incontinence can be difficult issues for both the prostate cancer survivor and their partner. It can be challenging to discuss these issues, but it's important to have open communication with your partner. Here are some tips for addressing sexual dysfunction and incontinence with your partner:

Be open and honest: It's important to have an open and honest conversation with your partner about the sexual side effects of prostate cancer treatment. Let them know how it's affecting you and how it makes you feel. This can help them understand what you're going through and how they can support you.

Educate your partner: Make sure your partner is informed about the sexual side effects of prostate cancer treatment. This will help them understand what's happening and how they can help.

Explore other ways of being intimate: There are many ways to be intimate besides sexual intercourse. Explore other forms of intimacy, such as cuddling, holding hands, or giving massages. This can help you maintain a close connection with your partner.

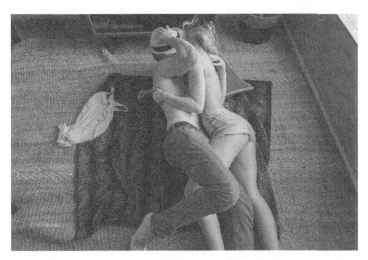

Try different positions: Experiment with different sexual positions that may be more comfortable and less likely to cause discomfort or pain.

Consider using aids: There are many aids available that can help with sexual dysfunction and incontinence. Talk to your healthcare provider about what might be appropriate for you and your partner.

Seek professional help: If sexual dysfunction or incontinence is causing significant distress, consider seeking professional help. A sex therapist or counselor can help you and your partner work through these issues and find ways to maintain intimacy and satisfaction in your relationship.

Chapter 5: Strategies for Improving Sexual Function and Intimacy

After prostate cancer treatment, many men experience sexual dysfunction that can impact their ability to have a fulfilling sex life. Fortunately, there are strategies that can help improve sexual function and quality of life. Here are some tips to consider:

Communicate with your partner: Open communication is key when dealing with sexual dysfunction. Talk to your partner about what you're going through and how you feel. Discuss ways to be intimate that don't involve intercourse.

Explore non-penetrative sexual activities: There are many non-penetrative sexual activities that can help maintain intimacy, such as cuddling, kissing, and sensual massage.

Try new positions: Experiment with different positions that are comfortable and put less pressure on the prostate.

Use lubrication: Lubrication can help reduce discomfort during sex.

Practice pelvic floor exercises: Pelvic floor exercises can help improve muscle tone and control, which can help improve erectile function.

Consider medication: There are medications available that can help improve erectile function, such as sildenafil (Viagra), tadalafil (Cialis), and vardenafil (Levitra).

Explore other treatments: There are other treatments available, such as penile injections, vacuum pumps, and penile implants. Discuss these options with your healthcare provider to determine if they may be right for you.

Remember, it's important to be patient and kind to yourself as you navigate this new chapter in your life. With time and the right strategies, you can improve your sexual function and enjoy intimacy once again.

Tips for enhancing intimacy after prostate cancer treatment

Prostate cancer and its treatment can affect sexual function and intimacy, but it's important to know that there are ways to improve and enhance intimacy after treatment. Here are some tips:

Be patient: It takes time to recover from prostate cancer treatment, and sexual function may not return to normal immediately. It's important to be patient and not rush things.

Communicate with your partner: Talking openly with your partner about your concerns, fears, and desires is important for maintaining intimacy. Your partner can also provide emotional support and encouragement.

Experiment with different positions: Trying different sexual positions can help you find what works best for you and your partner. It's important to communicate about what feels comfortable and what doesn't.

Use lubrication: Prostate cancer treatment can cause dryness and discomfort during sexual activity. Using lubrication can help alleviate this issue.

Practice Kegel exercises: Kegel exercises can help strengthen the pelvic floor muscles, which can improve sexual function and control over urinary incontinence.

Consider using aids: There are several aids available that can help improve sexual function and intimacy after prostate cancer treatment, such as penile implants, vacuum erection devices, and medication.

Remember, every person's experience with prostate cancer treatment is unique, and what works for one person may not work for another. It's important to talk to your healthcare provider about your concerns and explore your options for improving sexual function and intimacy after treatment.

Techniques for maintaining sexual health after prostate cancer treatment

Prostate cancer treatment can have a significant impact on sexual function, but there are several techniques that can be used to maintain sexual health after treatment. Here are some tips:

Pelvic floor exercises: Pelvic floor exercises can help improve urinary and sexual function after prostate cancer treatment. These exercises involve contracting and relaxing the muscles of the pelvic floor, which can help strengthen the muscles and improve control.

Vacuum erection device: A vacuum erection device is a non-invasive device that can be used to achieve and maintain an erection. The device works by creating a vacuum around the penis, which draws blood into the penis and causes an erection.

Medications: There are several medications that can be used to help improve erectile function after prostate cancer treatment. These medications work by increasing blood flow to the penis, which can help improve erections.

Penile injections: Penile injections involve injecting medication directly into the penis to help improve erectile function. This method can be effective for some men who have not responded to other treatments.

Sex therapy: Sex therapy can be helpful for couples who are struggling with sexual issues after prostate cancer treatment. A sex therapist can provide guidance on techniques for improving intimacy and communication, as well as help address any emotional or psychological issues related to sexual function.

It is important to remember that every person's experience with prostate cancer treatment is unique, and what works for one person may not work for another. It is important to work with a healthcare provider to determine the best course of action for maintaining sexual health after prostate cancer treatment.

Here are some additional techniques for maintaining sexual health after prostate cancer treatment:

Kegel exercises: These exercises strengthen the pelvic floor muscles that control urinary and ejaculatory function. They can be done discreetly anywhere and anytime and have been shown to improve urinary and sexual function after prostate cancer treatment.

Vacuum erection devices: These devices are used to create a vacuum around the penis, drawing blood into the shaft and causing an erection. They can be effective for men who experience erectile dysfunction after prostate cancer treatment and can be used in conjunction with other treatments like medications or injections.

Penile injections: These injections deliver medication directly into the penis to stimulate blood flow and create an erection. They can be effective for men who do not respond to oral medications like Viagra or Cialis.

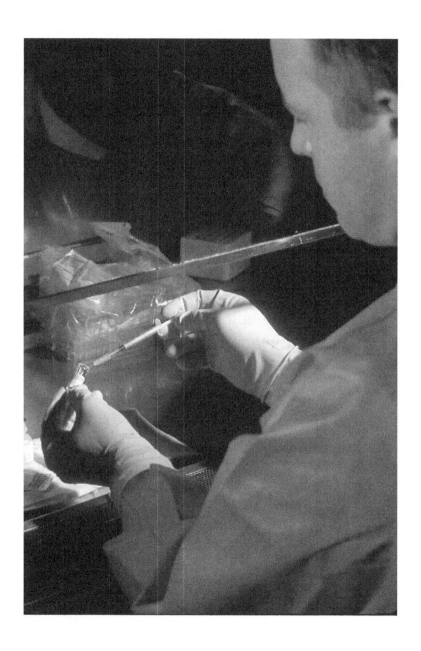

Testosterone replacement therapy: Some men may experience low testosterone levels after prostate cancer treatment, which can impact sexual function. Testosterone replacement therapy can be used to boost testosterone levels and improve libido and sexual function.

Penile implants: For men who do not respond to other treatments, penile implants may be an option. These devices are surgically implanted into the penis to create an erection on demand.

It's important to discuss all options with your healthcare provider and partner to determine the best approach for maintaining sexual health after prostate cancer treatment.

Chapter 6: Addressing Psychological Impacts on Sexual Health

The psychological impacts of prostate cancer on sexual health

Prostate cancer not only has physical impacts but can also have significant psychological impacts on a man's sexual health. The diagnosis of prostate cancer can be a traumatic experience, and undergoing treatment can be equally challenging. Many men may feel depressed, anxious, or angry, which can affect their sexual health and overall quality of life.

Depression is a common psychological effect of prostate cancer and can lead to a decreased interest in sexual activity. Anxiety can also play a role in sexual dysfunction by causing performance anxiety and inhibiting sexual arousal. Feelings of anger, frustration, and sadness may also impact a man's sexual health by reducing his desire for intimacy and leading to a sense of isolation.

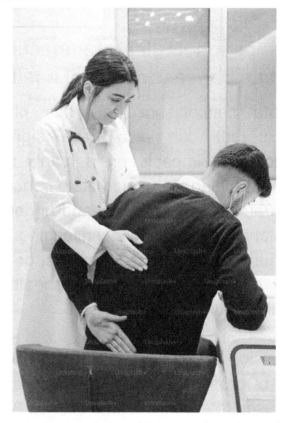

Moreover, prostate cancer treatment can cause physical changes that can further exacerbate the psychological impacts. For example, erectile dysfunction or incontinence can be very distressing for some men and may lead to feelings of inadequacy or embarrassment.

It is essential for men to acknowledge the psychological impact of prostate cancer on their sexual health and seek appropriate support. This support can include counseling, therapy, or support groups. Talking openly with a healthcare provider, partner, or counselor can help alleviate anxiety, depression, and other emotional issues related to prostate cancer and its treatment.

In conclusion, the psychological impact of prostate cancer on sexual health is significant and should not be overlooked. Men should seek support and talk about their emotional experiences to help them cope with the challenges of prostate cancer treatment and improve their sexual health and overall quality of life.

Coping with changes in sexual function after prostate cancer

Prostate cancer and its treatment can lead to changes in sexual function, which can be difficult to cope with for patients and their partners. Coping with these changes involves understanding the physical and emotional effects of the disease and taking steps to manage them. Here are some tips for coping with changes in sexual function after prostate cancer:

Communicate openly: Open and honest communication with your partner about your sexual function can help you both adjust to changes in your sex life. Talk about your concerns and feelings, and work together to find ways to maintain intimacy.

Seek support: Joining a support group for prostate cancer patients or speaking with a therapist can help you cope with the emotional impact of the disease and treatment. You may also benefit from talking with other couples who have experienced similar changes in their sex life.

Explore other forms of intimacy: Sexual intimacy is just one aspect of a relationship. Explore other ways to connect with your partner, such as cuddling, kissing, holding hands, or taking a walk together.

Learn about sexual aids: There are many products available to help manage changes in sexual function, such as erectile dysfunction medications, penile injections, and vacuum devices. Talk to your healthcare provider about what options may be right for you.

Focus on pleasure, not performance: It is important to shift the focus from achieving an erection or orgasm to simply enjoying physical intimacy and pleasure with your partner.

Stay physically active: Exercise can help improve overall health and sexual function. Talk to your healthcare provider about what types of exercise may be appropriate for you.

Adopt a healthy diet: A diet that is high in fruits, vegetables, and whole grains, and low in processed foods and saturated fats, can help maintain overall health and improve sexual function.

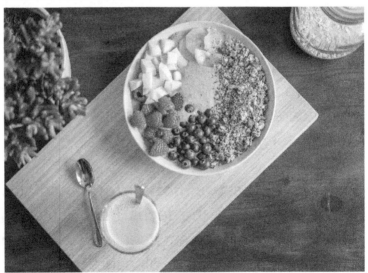

Remember that adjusting to changes in sexual function after prostate cancer is a process. It may take time to find new ways to be intimate with your partner, but with patience, communication, and a willingness to try new things, it is possible to maintain a fulfilling sex life.

Addressing emotional barriers to intimacy after prostate cancer

Addressing emotional barriers to intimacy after prostate cancer is an important step in overcoming the psychological impacts of prostate cancer on sexual health. Many men experience emotional barriers, such as anxiety, depression, and self-consciousness, that can affect their sexual relationships after treatment.

One of the most important things men can do is to talk to their partner openly and honestly about their feelings. It can be helpful to express concerns, such as feeling self-conscious about their body or their sexual performance. A partner who is informed and supportive can help to create a safe and supportive environment where both partners can feel comfortable and confident.

Men should also consider seeking professional counseling to address any emotional barriers they are facing. A counselor can help men to explore their feelings and develop coping strategies for dealing with anxiety, depression, and other emotional challenges. In some cases, couples counseling may also be beneficial, as it can help partners to communicate more effectively and work together to overcome any emotional barriers that may be impacting their sexual relationship.

Other strategies for addressing emotional barriers to intimacy after prostate cancer may include meditation, mindfulness, or other relaxation techniques. These practices can help men to reduce anxiety and stress, increase feelings of well-being and self-confidence, and create a more positive outlook on life.

Ultimately, the key to addressing emotional barriers to intimacy after prostate cancer is to be patient, open, and willing to communicate. By working together with a partner and seeking professional support when needed, men can overcome emotional barriers and enjoy fulfilling and satisfying sexual relationships.

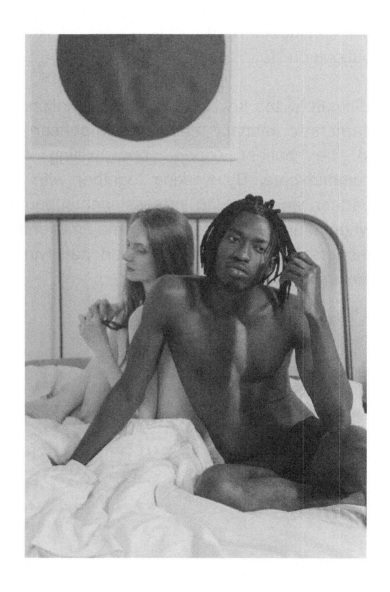

Chapter 7: Support for Partners of Prostate Cancer Survivors

Partners of prostate cancer survivors also face unique challenges and can benefit from support during and after their loved one's treatment. In many cases, partners may feel overwhelmed or uncertain about how to support their loved one, particularly in relation to sexual health and intimacy.

Here are some ways that partners can provide support:

Be informed: Educate yourself about prostate cancer, its treatments, and potential side effects, including those related to sexual function. This knowledge can help you better understand what your loved one is going through and how you can best support them.

Communicate openly: Encourage your loved one to talk about their feelings, concerns, and experiences related to their cancer diagnosis and treatment. Listen actively and without judgment, and offer reassurance and support.

Offer physical and emotional support: Physical touch, such as hugging or holding hands, can be comforting and reassuring. Additionally, offering emotional support through words of encouragement and affirmation can help your loved one feel loved and valued.

Attend appointments: Accompany your loved one to doctor's appointments, if possible, to provide emotional support and help ask questions and take notes.

Seek support for yourself: It's important to prioritize your own emotional well-being, as caring for a loved one with cancer can be emotionally taxing. Consider joining a support group for partners of cancer survivors, seeking therapy, or practicing self-care activities such as exercise, meditation, or journaling.

Remember, being a supportive partner mean you have to have all the answers or be perfect. Simply being present and showing that you care can make a significant difference in your loved one's journey towards recovery.

The impact of prostate cancer on partners

Prostate cancer not only affects the patient, but it can also have a significant impact on their partner. Partners may experience a range of emotions, such as anxiety, fear, and sadness, and may struggle to cope with the changes in their relationship and daily life.

Partners may feel a sense of helplessness, as they may not know how to best support their loved one through the diagnosis, treatment, and recovery process. They may also experience feelings of isolation, as they may not feel comfortable discussing their own emotions with their loved one or may not have a support network to turn to.

Furthermore, partners may also experience changes in their own sexual health, including a decreased desire for sex or difficulty achieving orgasm. This can add an additional layer of stress to an already challenging situation.

It is important for partners to recognize and address the impact that prostate cancer can have on their own emotional and physical well-being. By seeking support and communicating openly with their loved one and healthcare providers, partners can better cope with the challenges of prostate cancer and improve their overall quality of life.

Supporting partners through sexual dysfunction and incontinence

Prostate cancer not only affects the patient, but also their partner. Sexual dysfunction and incontinence can be difficult for both partners to cope with, and it's important for partners to receive support and understanding.

If your partner is experiencing sexual dysfunction or incontinence, it's important to understand that these are common side effects of prostate cancer treatment and are not their fault. You can provide support by actively listening to their concerns, being patient, and offering encouragement.

It's also important to remember that intimacy does not always have to involve sexual activity. You and your partner can still maintain intimacy through other means, such as cuddling, holding hands, or sharing hobbies and interests.

Encourage your partner to talk to their healthcare provider about their concerns and ask about potential treatments or therapies that may help improve their sexual function or incontinence. You can also attend appointments with your partner to provide emotional support and help ask questions.

Additionally, seeking support from a therapist or counselor can be helpful for both partners in coping with the emotional impacts of prostate cancer and its treatment on their relationship and sexual health. Support groups for couples affected by prostate cancer may also be available in your community or online.

Techniques for enhancing intimacy after prostate cancer

Intimacy after prostate cancer can be challenging, but it's still possible to maintain a fulfilling sex life. Here are some techniques for enhancing intimacy after prostate cancer:

Experiment with different sexual positions: Certain sexual positions may be more comfortable than others after prostate cancer treatment. Try different positions and find what works best for you and your partner.

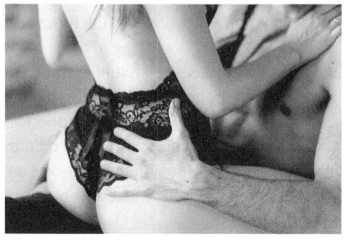

Use lubrication: Dryness and discomfort can be common issues after prostate cancer treatment. Using lubrication can help reduce friction and increase comfort during sexual activity.

Engage in non-sexual intimacy: Intimacy isn't just about sexual activity. Engaging in non-sexual intimacy, such as cuddling, kissing, and holding hands, can help maintain a connection with your partner.

Practice mindfulness: Mindfulness practices such as deep breathing, meditation, and yoga can help reduce stress and anxiety, which can improve overall sexual function.

Explore new forms of sexual expression: After prostate cancer treatment, you may need to explore new ways of experiencing sexual pleasure. Experiment with different forms of sexual expression such as oral sex, masturbation, and erotic massage.

Seek professional help: If you're experiencing difficulty with intimacy after prostate cancer, consider seeking the help of a therapist or sex therapist who specializes in sexual health issues. They can provide guidance and support as you navigate this challenging time.

Remember, every couple's experience with intimacy after prostate cancer will be different. It's important to communicate openly with your partner and find what works best for you both.

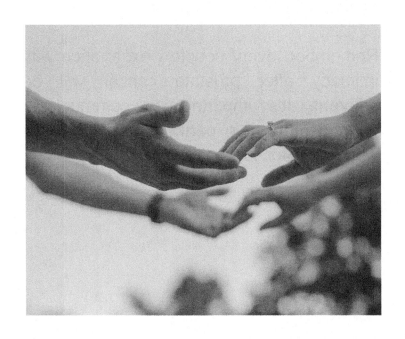

Chapter 8: Lifestyle Changes for Improved Sexual Health

Lifestyle changes can play an important role in maintaining and improving sexual health after prostate cancer treatment. Here are some strategies that can help:

Regular exercise: Exercise is not only good for your overall health but can also improve sexual function. Exercise can increase blood flow to the penis, which is essential for achieving and maintaining an erection. It can also reduce stress and anxiety, which can improve sexual function.

Healthy diet: A diet rich in fruits, vegetables, lean protein, and whole grains can help maintain a healthy weight and improve overall health, which can in turn improve sexual function.

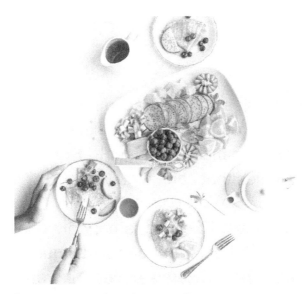

Stress reduction: Stress can have a negative impact on sexual function. Finding ways to reduce stress, such as meditation, deep breathing exercises, or yoga, can improve sexual function and overall well-being.

Quit smoking: Smoking can have a negative impact on blood flow and overall health, which can affect sexual function. Quitting smoking can improve overall health and sexual function.

Limit alcohol consumption: Alcohol can have a negative impact on sexual function. Limiting alcohol consumption can improve sexual function and overall health.

Get enough sleep: Lack of sleep can have a negative impact on sexual function. Getting enough sleep can improve sexual function and overall well-being.

Manage other health conditions: Managing other health conditions, such as diabetes and high blood pressure, can improve sexual function.

By implementing these lifestyle changes, prostate cancer survivors can improve their sexual health and overall well-being. It's important to talk to a healthcare provider before making any significant changes to your diet or exercise routine.

The role of lifestyle changes in improving sexual function

Lifestyle changes can play a crucial role in improving sexual function after prostate cancer treatment. Research has shown that making healthy lifestyle choices can help alleviate symptoms of sexual dysfunction and incontinence, and even improve overall sexual satisfaction. Here are some ways to improve your sexual health through lifestyle changes:

Exercise: Regular physical activity can improve cardiovascular health, increase energy levels, and help manage stress, all of which can contribute to improved sexual function. Kegel exercises, which target the pelvic floor muscles, can also help improve bladder control and sexual function.

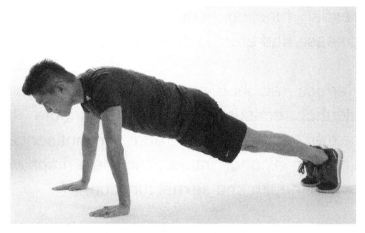

Nutrition: Eating a balanced diet that is rich in fruits, vegetables, whole grains, and lean protein can help support overall health and well-being. Some foods, such as those rich in antioxidants, may also have specific benefits for sexual health.

Weight management: Maintaining a healthy weight can help improve overall health and may reduce the risk of developing health conditions that can contribute to sexual dysfunction.

Quit smoking: Smoking can contribute to a range of health problems that can impact sexual function, such as cardiovascular disease and erectile dysfunction.

Reduce alcohol consumption: Excessive alcohol consumption can contribute to sexual dysfunction and incontinence. Limiting alcohol intake can help improve overall health and sexual function.

Manage stress: High levels of stress can impact sexual function and overall well-being. Techniques such as meditation, deep breathing, and yoga can help manage stress and improve sexual health.

Get enough sleep: Getting enough quality sleep is important for overall health and well-being, including sexual function. Aim for 7-9 hours of sleep each night.

By making these lifestyle changes, prostate cancer survivors can take an active role in improving their sexual health and overall well-being.

Dietary changes that may improve sexual health

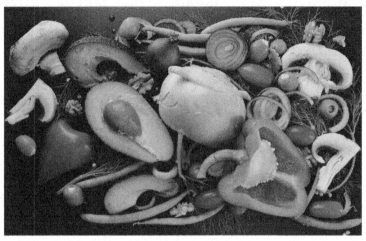

There are several dietary changes that may improve sexual health after prostate cancer treatment.

Consume more fruits and vegetables: Fruits and vegetables contain antioxidants, which can help reduce inflammation and oxidative stress in the body. This can improve blood flow to the genitals and may help improve sexual function.

Eat a diet rich in whole grains: Whole grains are rich in fiber and can help improve cardiovascular health. This can improve blood flow to the genitals, which may improve sexual function.

Incorporate healthy fats into your diet: Healthy fats, such as those found in fatty fish, nuts, and seeds, can help reduce inflammation and improve cardiovascular health. This can improve blood flow to the genitals and may improve sexual function.

Limit processed foods and sugar: Processed foods and sugar can contribute to inflammation in the body and can negatively impact cardiovascular health. This can lead to poor blood flow to the genitals and may contribute to sexual dysfunction.

Moderate alcohol consumption: Alcohol can have negative effects on sexual function.

Moderate alcohol consumption is defined as no more than two drinks per day for men.

It is important to note that dietary changes alone may not be enough to improve sexual function after prostate cancer treatment. It is important to discuss any concerns with your healthcare provider and work with a registered dietitian to develop a comprehensive plan for improving sexual health.

Exercise and sexual health

Exercise can play a significant role in improving sexual health in men. Regular physical activity has been linked to improved cardiovascular health, which can improve blood flow to the genitals and lead to stronger erections. Additionally, exercise can improve overall energy levels, which can enhance sexual desire and stamina.

Studies have also found that specific types of exercise, such as pelvic floor muscle exercises (also known as Kegels), can be particularly beneficial for men who have undergone prostate cancer treatment. These exercises can help strengthen the muscles that control urine flow and may also improve sexual function by increasing blood flow to the genitals.

It is important to note that men should consult with their healthcare provider before starting any new exercise regimen, particularly if they have undergone recent prostate cancer treatment or have other medical conditions that may affect their ability to exercise safely.

In addition to traditional exercise, engaging in regular sexual activity itself can also be a form of physical activity that can improve sexual health. Studies have found that men who have regular sexual activity have lower rates of erectile dysfunction and other sexual health problems.

Overall, incorporating regular physical activity and exercise into a healthy lifestyle can have a positive impact on sexual health in men.

Managing stress for improved sexual function

Stress can have a negative impact on many aspects of our health, including sexual function. It can cause fatigue, anxiety, and depression, which can all contribute to sexual dysfunction. Therefore, managing stress is an important part of maintaining and improving sexual health.

One effective way to manage stress is through relaxation techniques such as deep breathing, meditation, and yoga. These techniques can help reduce muscle tension, slow down breathing and heart rate, and promote a sense of calm and relaxation.

Regular exercise can also be an effective way to manage stress. Physical activity releases endorphins, which are natural mood-boosting chemicals in the brain that can help reduce stress and improve overall mood. Exercise can also improve circulation, which can benefit sexual function.

Other stress-reducing activities can include spending time in nature, engaging in creative hobbies, spending time with loved ones, and practicing self-care activities such as taking a warm bath or getting a massage.

In addition to managing stress, it's also important to address any underlying psychological issues that may be contributing to sexual dysfunction. Seeking support from a mental health professional can be helpful in managing these issues and improving sexual function.

Chapter 9: Alternative and Complementary Therapies

Alternative and complementary therapies are treatments that are used alongside traditional medical treatments for prostate cancer. These therapies aim to support the body's natural healing processes and may help alleviate symptoms of the disease or side effects of treatment. It is important to note that these therapies should not be used as a substitute for medical treatment and should always be discussed with a healthcare provider.

Here are some alternative and complementary therapies that have been studied for their potential benefits in managing prostate cancer and improving sexual function:

Acupuncture: Acupuncture is a traditional Chinese medicine technique that involves inserting thin needles into specific points on the body. Some studies have suggested that acupuncture may improve sexual function in men with prostate cancer who are experiencing erectile dysfunction.

Yoga: Yoga is a mind-body practice that involves physical postures, breathing exercises, and meditation. Some research has suggested that practicing yoga may improve sexual function and quality of life in men with prostate cancer.

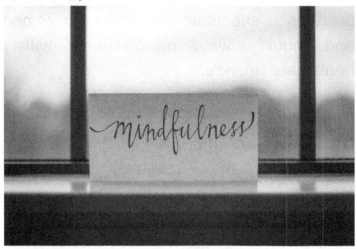

Massage therapy: Massage therapy involves manipulating the body's soft tissues to promote relaxation and relieve pain.

Some studies have suggested that massage therapy may improve sexual function in men with prostate cancer who are experiencing erectile dysfunction.

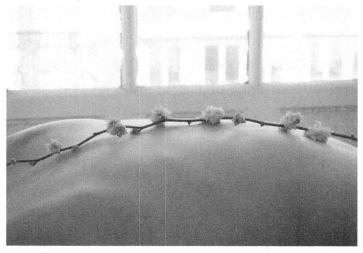

Herbal supplements: Some herbal supplements, such as ginseng and saw palmetto, have been studied for their potential benefits in managing prostate cancer and improving sexual function. However, it is important to note that the safety and effectiveness of these supplements have not been fully established and they can interact with other medications.

Mind-body techniques: Mind-body techniques, such as meditation and guided imagery, may help reduce stress and anxiety, which can have a positive impact on sexual function. Some studies have suggested that these techniques may also improve quality of life in men with prostate cancer.

It is important to note that while some alternative and complementary therapies may have potential benefits, others may be harmful or interfere with medical treatments. It is important to discuss any alternative therapies with a healthcare provider and to always follow their recommendations for managing prostate cancer and improving sexual health.

The role of alternative and complementary therapies in addressing sexual dysfunction

Alternative and complementary therapies are often used by prostate cancer survivors to improve sexual function after treatment. These therapies can be used in addition to traditional treatments or instead of them, depending on the individual's preferences and needs.

One alternative therapy that has shown some promise in improving sexual function is acupuncture. Acupuncture involves inserting small needles into specific points on the body to stimulate the flow of energy. Studies have shown that acupuncture can help to improve sexual function by increasing blood flow and reducing inflammation.

Another alternative therapy that may be helpful is herbal supplements. Certain herbs, such as ginseng and horny goat weed, have been used for centuries to improve sexual function. However, it is important to note that not all herbal supplements are safe or effective, and it is important to consult with a healthcare provider before taking any supplements.

Complementary therapies, such as yoga and meditation, may also be helpful in managing stress and improving sexual function. Yoga and meditation can help to reduce stress and anxiety, which are common contributors to sexual dysfunction.

It is important to note that alternative and complementary therapies should never be used as a substitute for traditional medical treatments. These therapies should always be used in conjunction with the guidance of a healthcare provider. Additionally, it is important to speak with a healthcare provider before beginning any new therapy to ensure that it is safe and appropriate for the individual's specific needs.

Acupuncture and sexual dysfunction

Acupuncture is an alternative therapy that has been used for thousands of years to treat a wide range of health conditions. It involves the insertion of thin needles into specific points on the body to stimulate the body's natural healing processes.

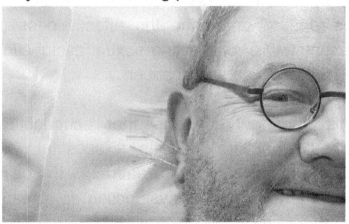

Acupuncture may be helpful in addressing sexual dysfunction in men who have undergone prostate cancer treatment. Some studies suggest that acupuncture can improve sexual function by increasing blood flow to the penis and reducing inflammation in the prostate.

In one study, men who received acupuncture reported significant improvements in erectile function, sexual desire, and overall sexual satisfaction compared to men who did not receive acupuncture. However, more research is needed to determine the effectiveness of acupuncture for treating sexual dysfunction in men with prostate cancer.

It's important to note that acupuncture should not be used as a substitute for conventional medical treatment. If you're experiencing sexual dysfunction as a result of prostate cancer treatment, be sure to talk to your healthcare provider about all of your treatment options, including alternative therapies like acupuncture.

Herbal remedies for improved sexual function

Herbal remedies have been used for centuries in traditional medicine to improve sexual function. While there is limited scientific research to support their effectiveness, some herbs are believed to have potential benefits for men with sexual dysfunction.

One of the most well-known herbs for sexual function is Panax ginseng, also known as Korean ginseng. This herb has been used in traditional medicine for centuries to treat a range of conditions, including erectile dysfunction. Some studies have suggested that Panax ginseng may help improve erectile function and sexual satisfaction in men.

Another herb that is sometimes used to improve sexual function is Tribulus terrestris. This plant has been used in traditional medicine to treat a variety of conditions, including sexual dysfunction. Some research has suggested that Tribulus terrestris may have a positive effect on sexual function in men with erectile dysfunction.

Other herbs that have been suggested as potential remedies for sexual dysfunction include horny goat weed, ginkgo biloba, and yohimbe. However, more research is needed to determine their effectiveness and safety.

It is important to note that herbal remedies can have side effects and can interact with other medications. Before using any herbal remedies for sexual dysfunction, it is important to talk to your healthcare provider to determine if they are safe for you and to ensure they do not interact with any medications you are taking.

Mind-body practices for enhancing sexual function

Mind-body practices can be effective in enhancing sexual function for prostate cancer survivors. These practices focus on the connection between the mind and body, and aim to promote relaxation, reduce stress, and improve overall well-being. Some of the most popular mind-body practices for enhancing sexual function include:

Meditation: Meditation is a relaxation technique that can help reduce stress, anxiety, and depression. Studies have shown that regular meditation can improve sexual function in both men and women.

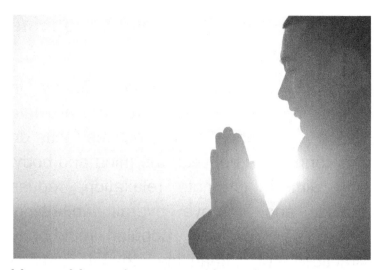

Yoga: Yoga is a practice that combines physical postures, breathing exercises, and meditation to promote relaxation and improve flexibility. Regular yoga practice has been shown to improve sexual function and reduce sexual dysfunction.

Tai chi: Tai chi is a gentle form of martial arts that involves slow, flowing movements and deep breathing. It has been shown to reduce stress, anxiety, and depression, and improve overall well-being, which can enhance sexual function.

Hypnotherapy: Hypnotherapy involves inducing a trance-like state to promote relaxation and reduce anxiety. It can be used to address psychological issues related to sexual function, such as anxiety, performance anxiety, and negative self-talk.

Cognitive-behavioral therapy (CBT): CBT is a type of therapy that helps individuals identify and change negative thought patterns and behaviors. It can be effective in addressing psychological issues related to sexual function, such as anxiety, depression, and negative self-talk.

It is important to note that while these mind-body practices can be helpful in enhancing sexual function, they should not be used as a replacement for medical treatment or advice. It is always important to consult with a healthcare provider before starting any new therapy or practice.

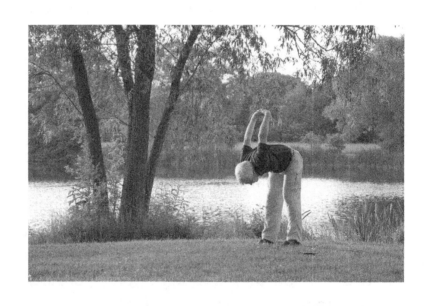

Chapter 10: Moving Forward: Life After Prostate Cancer

Adjusting to life after prostate cancer treatment

Adjusting to life after prostate cancer treatment can be challenging for many survivors. After undergoing treatment, individuals may experience a range of physical, emotional, and psychological changes that can affect their quality of life. It is important to take time to adjust to these changes and find ways to cope with them effectively.

One of the most common challenges faced by prostate cancer survivors is sexual dysfunction. This can include erectile dysfunction, loss of libido, and difficulty achieving orgasm. Other common side effects of prostate cancer treatment include fatigue, incontinence, and changes in bowel habits.

In addition to physical changes, survivors may also experience emotional and psychological changes. Many men report feeling anxious or depressed after treatment, and some may struggle with feelings of anger, frustration, or sadness.

To adjust to life after prostate cancer treatment, it can be helpful to take a holistic approach that addresses both the physical and emotional aspects of recovery. This may include:

Seeking support: Joining a support group for prostate cancer survivors can be an effective way to connect with others who have gone through similar experiences. Talking to others who understand what you are going through can help reduce feelings of isolation and provide a sense of community.

Seeking professional support: If you are struggling with anxiety, depression, or other emotional issues, it may be helpful to seek the support of a mental health professional. A therapist can help you develop coping strategies and provide support as you adjust to life after treatment.

Engaging in physical activity: Exercise can help reduce fatigue, improve mood, and enhance overall physical health. Talk to your healthcare provider about developing an exercise plan that is safe and appropriate for your individual needs.

Eating a healthy diet: A healthy diet can help support overall health and well-being. Talk to your healthcare provider or a registered dietitian about developing a nutrition plan that is tailored to your individual needs.

Exploring complementary therapies: Some survivors may find that complementary therapies, such as acupuncture, massage, or meditation, can help reduce stress and improve overall well-being.

Finding ways to maintain intimacy: Although sexual dysfunction can be a challenging side effect of prostate cancer treatment, it is important to find ways to maintain intimacy with your partner. This may include exploring non-sexual forms of intimacy, such as cuddling or holding hands, or working with a healthcare provider or therapist to develop strategies for managing sexual dysfunction.

Taking time to adjust: Adjusting to life after prostate cancer treatment takes time, and it is important to be patient with yourself as you navigate this process. Be kind to yourself, and seek support when you need it. Remember that recovery is a journey, and that with time and effort, you can adapt to the changes in your life and find ways to live a fulfilling and meaningful life after treatment.

Finding new ways to experience pleasure and intimacy

After prostate cancer treatment, some men may find that their sexual function has changed, and it may take some time to adjust to these changes. However, it's important to note that pleasure and intimacy can still be experienced in different ways. Here are some ideas for finding new ways to experience pleasure and intimacy after prostate cancer treatment:

Explore other erogenous zones: While the penis may no longer be a primary source of sexual pleasure, other areas of the body, such as the nipples, ears, neck, and inner thighs, can still be sensitive and pleasurable.

Experiment with different types of touch: Try using different types of touch, such as light touch, deep pressure, or vibrations, to find what feels good.

Engage in non-sexual intimacy: Cuddling, holding hands, kissing, and spending time together can all help to create intimacy and closeness.

Experiment with different sexual positions: Trying out different positions can help to find what is comfortable and pleasurable.

Use sex toys: Sex toys can be a great way to explore new sensations and experiences.

Communicate with your partner: Talking openly and honestly with your partner about your needs, desires, and limitations can help to strengthen your relationship and find new ways to experience pleasure together.

Remember, the most important thing is to approach intimacy and sexual pleasure with an open mind and a willingness to try new things. With patience, experimentation, and communication, it is possible to find new ways to experience pleasure and intimacy after prostate cancer treatment.

Embracing a new normal

Embracing a new normal can be a difficult task, especially for prostate cancer survivors who have undergone treatment and may have experienced changes in their sexual function. However, it is important to remember that adjusting to a new normal is a process that takes time, patience, and effort.

One way to begin the process of embracing a new normal is to focus on the positive changes that have occurred in your life as a result of your treatment. Perhaps you have developed a new appreciation for life, or have become more mindful of your health and well-being. Take some time to reflect on these positive changes and use them as motivation to move forward.

It can also be helpful to set new goals and priorities for yourself. This can give you a sense of purpose and direction as you navigate your post-treatment life. Whether it is pursuing a new hobby, setting a fitness goal, or volunteering for a cause you care about, finding something to work towards can help you feel empowered and in control.

It is important to remember that adjusting to a new normal can be an ongoing process, and that it is okay to ask for help along the way. This may include seeking support from loved ones, joining a support group for prostate cancer survivors, or seeking professional help from a therapist or counselor.

Ultimately, the key to embracing a new normal after prostate cancer treatment is to stay positive, stay motivated, and stay connected to your support network. By doing so, you can continue to find joy and fulfillment in your life, even in the face of adversity.

Looking for more information on the diagnosis, treatment, and recovery process for prostate cancer? Check out our companion guide, Prostate Cancer: From Diagnosis to Recovery, which provides in-depth insights and practical advice for men and their loved ones facing prostate cancer. Click here to access the book and learn more about navigating the prostate cancer journey."

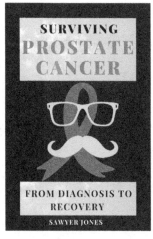 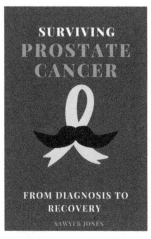

Kindle version   Paperback version

You can also click on the images and it will direct you to the book.

Conclusion

Prostate cancer and its treatments can have significant impacts on sexual health and function, but there are many ways to address these challenges and improve intimacy and sexual satisfaction after treatment. Communication with healthcare providers and partners is crucial, as is a willingness to explore new techniques and approaches. Lifestyle changes such as exercise and stress reduction, as well as alternative therapies like acupuncture and herbal remedies, may also help improve sexual function. Ultimately, embracing a new normal and finding new ways to experience pleasure and intimacy can help prostate cancer survivors and their partners navigate the challenges of life after treatment and enjoy a fulfilling sex life.

Encouragement to prioritize sexual health after prostate cancer.

As we conclude, it's essential to remind those who have gone through prostate cancer treatment and their partners that it's crucial to prioritize sexual health. The journey to recovery from prostate cancer treatment can be challenging, but it's important to remember that there is life after the diagnosis, and you can still have a fulfilling sex life. Remember that sexual health is not only physical but also emotional and psychological. Therefore, it's crucial to communicate effectively with your healthcare provider about any concerns regarding sexual health.

Additionally, don't hesitate to reach out for support from family, friends, or a support group. There are resources available to help you and your partner navigate the challenges that come with prostate cancer treatment. Embracing a new normal may not be easy, but with time, patience, and understanding, you can adjust and enjoy a fulfilling sex life.

In conclusion, prioritize your sexual health after prostate cancer treatment, embrace the changes, communicate openly, and explore different options for enhancing intimacy. Remember that you are not alone, and there is support available to help you navigate this journey.

Made in the USA
Las Vegas, NV
05 September 2023

77126149R00069